Enjoy
great sleep

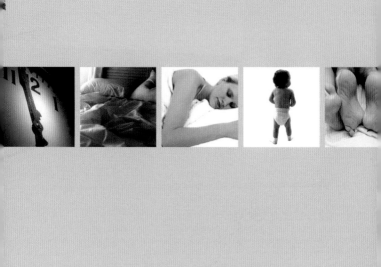

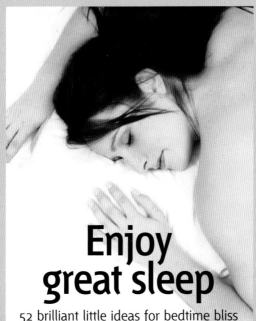

Enjoy
great sleep

52 brilliant little ideas for bedtime bliss

Karen Williamson

brilliantideas

CAREFUL NOW

Follow the tips in this book and
you could soon be well on your
way to blissful sleep every
night. Please remember that
any advice given in this book
is not a substitute for medical
advice – so consult your doctor
or healthcare provider before
making any changes to your
diet and exercise regime or if
you start taking supplements –
particularly if you're on
medication, you're very unfit or
you're pregnant. And don't
forget that how well you sleep
is ultimately up to you.

Copyright © The Infinite Ideas Company Ltd, 2007

The right of Karen Williamson to be identified as the
author of this book has been asserted in accordance
with the Copyright, Designs and Patents Act 1988.

First published in 2007 by
The Infinite Ideas Company Limited
36 St Giles
Oxford, OX1 3LD
United Kingdom
www.infideas.com

All rights reserved. Except for the quotation of small
passages for the purposes of criticism or review, no part
of this publication may be reproduced, stored in a
retrieval system or transmitted in any form or by any
means, electronic, mechanical, photocopying, recording,
scanning or otherwise, except under the terms of the
Copyright, Designs and Patents Act 1988 or under the
terms of a licence issued by the Copyright Licensing
Agency Ltd, 90 Tottenham Court Road, London W1T 4LP,
UK, without the permission in writing of the publisher.
Requests to the publisher should be addressed to the
Permissions Department, Infinite Ideas Limited, 36 St
Giles, Oxford, OX1 3LD, UK, or faxed to +44 (0)1865
514777.

A CIP catalogue record for this book is available from the
British Library
ISBN 978-1-905940-18-9

Brand and product names are trademarks or registered
trademarks of their respective owners..

Designed and typeset by Baseline Arts Ltd, Oxford
Printed in China

Brilliant ideas

Introduction

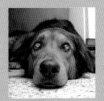

You don't really question sleep until you're not getting enough. And it's only when symptoms spiral out of control that you think about doing anything. Suddenly you're falling asleep during conversations, unable to concentrate on anything longer than an ad break on TV, can't be bothered to socialise any more and it's the fourth time this week you've put the tea bag in cold water. Even then, it often takes a comment from someone else – 'Gosh you've been looking tired lately', 'You're not as lively as you used to be', or 'If you don't do something about your snoring, I'm going to leave you' – before you actually decide to take action.

The fact is, there are some pretty straightforward strategies to help you get the sleep you deserve. Just understanding what happens to your body while you sleep will help you work out the mechanisms behind your sleep problems – whether it's insomnia, nightmares, restless legs syndrome or sleep apnea. And finding out about your body clock means you won't waste time trying out things that won't ever work. If you're a night owl, for instance, there's no point going to bed at 10pm – you'll be staring at the ceiling for 5 hours, churning over your thoughts. By the time you're ready to drop off, you'll have convinced yourself that you're going to get the sack, die horribly on your cycle ride to work or be abandoned by your partner.

The key to solving your sleep problem is finding the cause – be it stress, bad diet, lack of exercise or a noisy bedroom environment – and being persistent. That means not giving up if the first thing you try doesn't work. I've come up with a huge selection of tried-and-tested solutions so I guarantee you won't run out of things to try – from changing your bedtime routine and visualisation tricks to decluttering your bedroom and performing wake-me-up morning stretches.

Try everything that takes your fancy, write down how well it worked, keep referring back to your notes and soon you should have a list of all those changes you've made that do the trick. It may take one week or it may take a few months. But don't give up. Before you know it, you'll be sleeping soundly every night, waking up in a great mood and managing to stay fully awake during every conversation you have in the day.

1. Eyes wide shut

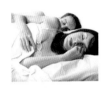

We spend a third of our lives asleep – so what actually happens to our body when we're tucked up under the duvet?

Sleep takes place in cycles, each lasting around 60 minutes in babies and 90 minutes in adults. During a night, a normal sleeper can expect to go through 4–5 cycles. And each sleep cycle goes through 5 stages of sleep. The body is thought to repair and regenerate itself in the first 4 stages of sleep – commonly known as non-REM sleep (NREM). Stage 5, REM (Rapid eye movement) sleep, is where the brain sorts out and makes sense of the events of the day – it's also when you're most likely to dream.

Stage 1
Light sleep Heart rate and body temperature drop and brain waves slow down even more. It lasts a few minutes and you can easily be woken up during this stage.

Stage 2
Proper sleep This phase usually lasts about 30–40 minutes and although it doesn't take much to wake you up, you're likely to feel groggy.

Defining idea

'Life is something you do when you can't get to sleep.'
FRAN LEBOWITZ, US writer

Stages 3 and 4

Deep sleep In stage 3, brainwaves give way to the slowest brain waves – the delta waves. By stage 4, not much is going to wake you. Your oxygen levels, heart rate and breathing levels are at their lowest. Now growth hormone is released, which helps cell renewal, building and repairing body tissue.

Stage 5

This is when you have your most vivid dreams, and your body and brain come to life – your brain is as active as it is when you're awake but apart from finger and facial twitching, most of your muscles become paralysed to stop you acting out your dreams. Your eyes dart about, while your heart rate, breathing rate and blood pressure all rise and can be erratic. Your memory is also being recharged.

The exact pattern varies from person to person and with age. Babies spend about half their sleeping time in REM sleep, adults about a quarter. If you miss out on sleep, it's the lighter stages of sleep that tend to be lost. The body will always do its best to catch up on deep sleep first, then REM sleep.

2. Rhythms of life

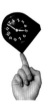

Understand your body clock – and determine all your energy highs and lows in the day.

Your body clock normally works to a daily 24-hour cycle – and controls the release of hormones, blood pressure and heart rate plus when your body wants to go to sleep and wake up. We're programmed to fall asleep at night, when it's dark and cooler, and to be awake when it's light and warmer. Your body clock controls your temperature and sleepiness so that at night your temperature drops as you go to sleep and rises as you wake. It also makes sure you don't have inconvenient needs – like going to the toilet or feeling hungry. You have another drop in temperature and sleepiness around midday until two in the afternoon.

In the morning light enters the eye and hits the retina. This travels along nerves and ends up in a part of your brain responsible for regulating your body clock. Here signals are sent to the pineal gland in your brain to stop producing melatonin, the brain's sleep-

Here's an idea for you

Your body clock also controls your day's movements – over 24 hours, you get restless and need a change of pace every 90 to 120 minutes. Observe these changes one day – see how you get up from your desk, stretch, have a cup of coffee, then get back to work, stop for lunch, have a cup of tea and so on.

Defining idea

'Sleeping is no mean art: for its sake
one must stay awake all day'
FRIEDRICH NIETZSCHE

inducing hormone and to release
the get-up-and-go hormone
cortisol. In the evening the fading
light of the setting sun triggers
melatonin to prepare your body for
sleep. Once you're asleep, if you
suddenly put on a light – to go to the toilet, for instance – chances are
you'll have trouble dropping off again, because light kick-starts those
get-up-and-go hormones, and as far as they're concerned it's wake-up
time. The average body clock is happiest when you sleep from around
11pm to 7am, which is when all the hormones are programmed to be
either released or stopped.

Some studies suggest that the hormone melatonin, given as a
supplement at specific times, may be useful for resetting daily
rhythms to help overcome the effects of jet lag and sleep disorders.

3. Lark or owl?

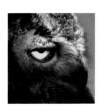

Do your eyelids start drooping after the early evening news or are you doing the mamba at midnight?

Some people's body clocks are slightly out of sync with the 24 hour pattern. 'Owls' have a longer daily cycle and a slower body clock, they want to go to bed later and are slow to get going in the morning. Owls often have trouble getting to sleep and stay in light sleep longer. The body clocks of 'larks' run slightly faster than average and their daily cycle is slightly shorter. So larks want to go to bed early, get up early and are irritatingly bright eyed and bushy tailed the minute they get up.

Generally we become more owl-like when we're teenagers and more lark-like when we get older. If you are either of these types, there's not much you can do to change it, but there are tricks to help you adapt.

If you're a **lark** who wants to stay up later, spend time outside in the afternoon or early evening. Then go for a brisk walk or do some light

Here's an idea for you

Write a list of which time in the day you are most alert and most productive. If you're a lark, it'll be some time between late morning and noon. If you're an owl, you'll get a short burst of productivity late morning, but you'll feel most alert around 6pm. Then tailor your most challenging tasks around your up times.

Defining idea

'Early to rise, and early to bed, makes a man healthy, wealthy and dead.'
JAMES THURBER

stretching. Sleep with curtains closed and, if you want to stay up later more regularly, consider buying black-out curtains which block out the light. Darkness tells your brain it's time to sleep.

If you're an **owl** who wants to be more alert in the morning, keep your evenings quiet to help prepare your body for bed, sleep with curtains open and let daylight wake you up naturally. Walk outside as soon as possible after waking up. You should also do as much as you can the night before, select the next day's clothes for instance, so you don't have to think too hard in the morning.

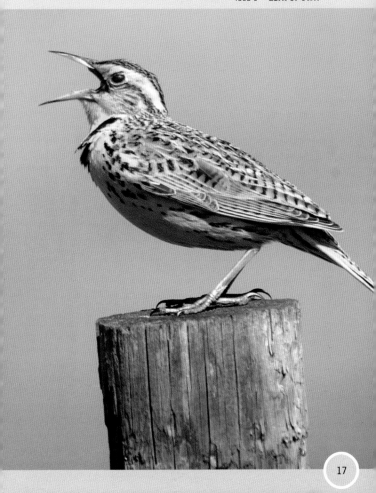

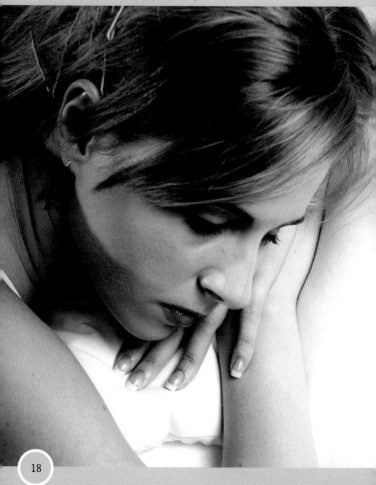

4. System failure

**Injury, poor performance and depression –
the results of not getting your sleep
quota**

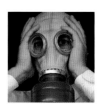

During a good night's sleep, in the REM stage, the brain busily
replenishes the neurotransmitters that organise neural networks
vital for remembering, learning, performance and problem solving.
If you deprive the brain of sleep, you get less REM sleep and your
memory will be poorer.

Studies show that sleep deprivation can severely affect driving
ability. One comparing the reaction times between people who were
sleep deprived and those who'd been drinking alcohol suggested
that driving when tired is as dangerous as driving drunk.

Recent research demonstrated that
the nightly loss of four hours of
sleep over 10 days in healthy young
adults significantly reduced their
immune function. The number of
white blood cells and their activity
was decreased. Missing sleep can
actually speed up aging. Sleeping

Here's an idea for you

Set yourself a test to find how lack of
sleep affects you. Write down the
names of 10 random objects which you
then need to recall on another piece of
paper. Time yourself when you do the
test feeling rested, and compare the
results after doing it again (with a new
list) when you're sleep deprived.

for only four hours a night for as little as a week, reduces the body's ability to process and store carbohydrates and regulate hormone levels – changes which are similar to those of advanced ageing.

Lack of sleep makes you hungry and more prone to putting on weight. The key to this is the hormone leptin, which signals when the body needs or does not need more food. Leptin levels rise during sleep and this tells your brain that you've eaten enough; when you're sleep deprived, leptin levels are low, so your brain thinks you need to eat more. Research has also shown that insufficient sleep impairs the body's ability to use insulin, which can lead to the onset of diabetes.

Blood pressure usually falls during the sleep cycle, but interrupted sleep can adversely affect this normal decline, leading to hypertension and cardiovascular problems. One study of nurses showed that those sleeping five hours or less had a 45 per cent greater risk of developing heart disease than those sleeping eight hours.

5. Six, seven or eight?

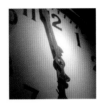

How much sleep you really need?

Sleep experts don't normally talk in terms of number of hours, but the amount of sleep you need to be wide awake and alert in the day. So if you regularly fall asleep watching TV or reading or fall asleep in the car, you might not be getting enough.

That said, women seem to need about 20 minutes sleep more than men. The experts say it's because women use their brains in a more flexible way than men – which means their brains are working harder in the day and are therefore more tired at night.

In general the amount of sleep needed decreases with age. By the time you're 60 you'll probably only need 5 or 6 hours a night. The amount of slow wave sleep, which is when the human growth hormone is secreted, is much higher in children and decreases with age. A teenager's body clock actually resets so instead of

Here's an idea for you

To find out how many hours of sleep you need record the amount and quality of sleep you had during the night and rate your daytime functioning at the end of the day on a scale from 1 (unable to think straight, constantly tired) to 10 (perfect performance). After two weeks, look at the results and work out in what way your sleep relates to how you function the next day.

Defining idea

'A satisfying sleep, like a satisfying meal, can leave one happy and content, without feeling too full, and with room, perhaps, for just a little more'
Sleep expert JIM HORNE

producing the sleep-inducing melatonin earlier in the evening – like kids and adults – their body's not triggering it until 1 in the morning. So the average teenager would be much happier waking up at around 10.

If you want to increase the amount of time you're asleep, don't suddenly go to bed an hour earlier than usual – you'll just lie awake in bed. Just go to bed 10 to 15 minutes earlier than usual every night until you're waking up refreshed. Then stick to this bedtime as much as possible so your body knows when to prepare for sleep.

6. The big one

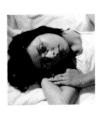

Can't get to sleep or keep waking up? Chances are, you've got insomnia – the biggest cause of sleep problems.

Insomnia is when you're not getting enough uninterrupted sleep to leave you refreshed the next day. The reasons we have trouble sleeping vary from anxiety (e.g. over work) to physical illness, depression or a sleep disorder such as sleep apnea. The majority of insomnia will only last for a few nights and is caused by some change to your sleep schedule such as jet lag, illness or a forthcoming big event, and once this has gone, your sleep will go back to normal. Women may suffer disturbed sleep during a period. Short term insomnia will last three to four weeks but if the cause is not addresses it can lead to chronic insomnia, which lasts over a month, occurring every night or every now and then.

Normal sleepers take less than 20 minutes to fall asleep – if you're the type of insomniac who can't get to sleep it could take more than 30

Here's an idea for you

Keep a sleep diary for three weeks. Write down how long it takes to get to sleep, how many times you wake up during the night and what time you wake up in the morning – plus how you feel the next day. After a few weeks you should see a pattern emerging. Now you can start to find solutions..

Defining idea

'Perhaps that's why some of us are insomniacs; night is so precious that it would be pusillanimous to sleep all through it!'
Sci fi author BRIAN W. ALDISS

minutes no matter how tired you are. This is often due to anxiety, but it could be that your body clock is running too late.

Everyone wakes up momentarily throughout the night, but we're not aware of it so it doesn't affect our sleep. Some insomniacs, however, wake up in the middle of the night, and spend what seems like ages, tossing and turning. You can be awake for hours or just wake up frequently. Triggers include snoring, sleep apnea or sometimes depression.

If you've got early morning insomnia you'll wake up more than an hour before you want to. Depression or a body that's set to wake up too early are common causes.

7. Back to basics

**Your first steps in beating insomnia –
time to reset your body clock.**

There's no point being in bed if you're not
asleep – you'll just start associating bed with being awake. If you
don't go to bed until you're really tired and get up early, the theory
is you'll drop off more quickly, have less interrupted sleep and more
deep sleep.

Sleep efficiency is the percentage of time you spend in bed asleep. A
good sleeper will have sleep efficiency of around 90 per cent. If you
have 70 per cent or less, think about reducing the time you spend in
bed so that it more closely matches the time you're asleep.

To decide when to go bed keep a sleep diary for a week to work out
how much sleep on average you're
getting a night. Once you've got a
figure, add one hour then work
backwards from the time you need
to get up to calculate your bedtime.
You shouldn't spend under 5 and a
half hours in bed – the average
basic sleep requirement.

Here's an idea for you

To work out your sleep efficiency – the
amount of time in bed actually asleep,
you divide the time spent asleep by the
time spent in bed and multiply this by
100. If you slept for 6 hours but were
in bed for 9, your sleep efficiency is 66
per cent.

25

Defining idea

'If you can't sleep, then get up and do something instead of lying there worrying. It's the worry that gets you, not the lack of sleep.'
DALE CARNEGIE, self-help guru

Once your sleep efficiency has improved to about 85 per cent for two weeks, you can increase your time in bed by 15 minutes a week by going to bed 15 minutes earlier but getting up at the same time until you've increased your sleeping time enough to feel good and function well during the day.

If you do wake in the night, get up, go into another room and do something like listening to relaxing music, reading or relaxation exercises – don't watch TV or surf the net. When your eyelids start to droop, then return to your bed.

8. Wired!

How tea, coffee, alcohol and other stimulants can play havoc with your sleep cycle.

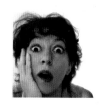

Caffeine stimulates the central nervous system, increasing your metabolic rate, blood pressure, heart rate, and breathing levels and its effects can last longer than four hours. Having a caffeinated drink at night is particularly thought to disturb deep sleep and REM sleep. Limit yourself to two cups of coffee or four of tea daily, but don't have them too late in the day. Try decaffeinated versions or other drinks such as herbal teas, water and fruit juice instead. If you're relying on coffee to give you energy, try snacks such as a banana, dried fruit or a cereal bar instead.

Although it's a sedative, alcohol causes the release of adrenaline and blocks tryptophan, which helps the body make the calming brain chemical serotonin – vital for sleep. One unit of alcohol takes about one hour to metabolise. So if you drink three glasses of wine at 10pm, expect your sleep to be disrupted from around 1am. Try to have at

Here's an idea for you

If you want to drink less alcohol at home, use a tall, slim glass. Research has shown that that we serve ourselves 20 per cent more when using a short, wide glass than when the glass is tall and slim.

Defining idea

'I always keep a stimulant handy in case I see a snake, which I also keep handy.'
W.C. FIELDS

least two drink-free days a week and don't drink more than two units of alcohol per day if you're a women, three units if you're a man. Sip drinks slowly so they lasts longer and try to eat before you start drinking since it will help reduce the amount of alcohol absorbed by your body.

You may think nicotine relaxes you but it can cause difficulty falling asleep, problems waking in the morning, and even nightmares. So bite the bullet and quit. If you're a woman, you're much more likely to succeed if you do it in the first half of your menstrual cycle because nicotine withdrawal symptoms – depression, anxiety and irritability – are worse in the second half. There's a host of options to help you quit, from nicotine patches and self-help manuals to acupuncture and hypnotherapy.

9. Noisy nights!

Stop snoring before it ruins your sleep – and your relationship

Find the cause of your snoring and tackle it:

Find out if you're overweight by checking your Body Mass Index (BMI). Divide your weight (kg) by your height squared (m). If your BMI is greater than 25 you are overweight. If your collar size is over 16.5 inches you're likely to snore because the muscles around your windpipe can't support the fat around it when you're asleep. Even a small loss of weight can improve symptoms.

Cigarette smoke irritates the lining of the nasal cavity and throat causing swelling and catarrh. If the nasal passages become congested it's difficult to breathe through your nose because there's less airflow. The more you smoke, the worse your snoring. Until you quit try to give up smoking at least 4 hours before bed. Drinking triggers snoring as it reduces the tone of

Here's an idea for you

Sleeping on your back can cause snoring as it allows the flesh of your throat to relax and block airways. If your snoring is made worse by sleeping on your back and you're finding it impossible to sleep on your side, try sewing a tennis ball into the back of your pyjamas, which will make it impossible to sleep on your back.

Defining idea

'I think a woman married to a snorer should be granted a divorce without any argument'
H V MORTON, travel writer (1892 – 1979)

the muscles that keep the upper breathing passage open. So keep to the limit and avoid drinking just before bedtime.

If you can only snore with your mouth open then you are a 'mouth breather'. You'll probably wake up with a dry mouth and sometimes a sore throat because of the strain of snoring. When we breathe in through the mouth the air hitting the back of the throat can create enormous vibrations in the soft tissue. Try to breathe through your nose – and ask your pharmacist for gadgets (such as chin strips) that help keep your mouth closed. To help clear your nose, put a few drops of eucalyptus on your pillowcase. Small or collapsing nostrils can prevent you from breathing through your nose. Try nasal strips which you place on the outside of the nostrils to stop them collapsing.

10. Snores you can't ignore

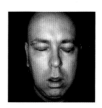

When snoring gets serious and breathing stops – that's sleep apnea.

Your snoring could be a problem if you have loud, frequent bursts of snoring followed by quiet periods then a sudden gasping for air. These periods of silence mean that you're not breathing and can last from 10 seconds to as long as two minutes. This can happen hundreds of times a night although you'll have no recollection of it the next morning.

What happens is that your throat closes and you cannot suck air into your lungs. This is because the muscles that hold your throat open when you're awake relax during sleep and allow it to narrow. So when your throat is partially closed or the muscles relax too much, every time you inhale you'll suck your throat until it's completely closed and air won't be able to pass at all. Rising

Here's an idea for you

To help you understand what happens during an episode of sleep apnea put your hand over your vacuum cleaner intake nozzle. Your hand blocks all air from getting through even though the vacuum cleaner is still applying suction, in the same way that we still try to breathe. The vacuum cleaner will be straining now – just as your body would be.

Defining idea

'Laugh and the world laughs with you. Snore and you sleep alone.'
ANTHONY BURGESS

carbon dioxide levels wake you up slightly, and this sends a signal from the brain to the throat muscles that enlarge the airway to open up – so breathing starts again, often with a loud snort or gasp.

When you stop breathing, the level of oxygen in the blood goes down and the level of carbon dioxide goes up, forcing the heart to work harder, changing your heart rate and even increasing blood pressure. The rise in carbon dioxide levels also affects circulation, particularly in your brain. If you're regularly waking up with headaches, this may be why.

As with snoring, smoking, drinking alcohol and being overweight can bring on sleep apnea. It's common during pregnancy when it has to be treated seriously as it can affect the baby. Sleep apnea can also be caused by a blockage in the nose or throat such as a short jaw, large tonsils, swollen nasal passages from allergies or a tongue that is too far back.

11. Breathe easy

All you need to know about putting a stop to sleep apnea

So you think you might have sleep apnea? See
your doctor and bring along your regular sleeping partner, if you
have one. Your doctor will ask about sleep and daytime sleepiness.
She will look for abnormalities in your breathing passage such as a
crooked nose or enlarged tonsils and may order blood tests to
ensure your respiratory system and heart are normal. You may then
be referred to a sleep disorders clinic for overnight testing. Once
diagnosed try some of the ideas below.

Being overweight can make it more
difficult to breathe when you're
asleep. The best way to slim down
for good is to lose no more than 2lb
a week on a low-fat diet with
plenty of fruit and vegetables. This
demands willpower and a
completely new approach to
eating. Giving up smoking will
return lung capacity to normal,
making breathing easier. Don't

Here's an idea for you

If you need to lose weight to help you
breathe more easily at night, try one of
the following psychological tricks to help
you stick to your healthy eating plan.
Stick an old picture of you when you
were slimmer on the fridge to put you in
the right frame of mind when you open
it. Alternatively, a photo of you on the
beach during your last holiday may make
you more likely to grab the salad rather
than the cheese cake.

drink alcohol or take sleeping tablets, both of which depress your breathing reflexes. Try aromatherapy: put a few drops of olbas, eucalyptus or peppermint oil in a diffuser at night.

Your dentist can fit an oral appliance which brings your tongue and lower jaw forward, therefore widening the airway. Continuous positive airway pressure (CPAP) is currently the most successful treatment. When you're asleep you wear a mask over your nose, which blows air into it through a tube. This is connected to a small device which generates enough pressure to keep your airway from collapsing and open your breathing passage.

If the obstruction is caused by an abnormality in your nose or throat, then you may need surgery to fix it. The success rate, however, is only about 50 per cent.

12. Sleep attack

The ins and outs of narcolepsy.

Narcolepsy is a sleep disorder which makes you fall asleep at inappropriate times and places. It can begin at any age but once you've got it, you've got it for life. Sufferers are often very sleepy most of the time, but then have trouble falling asleep at night. As soon as they drop off, or start to wake up, they can have vivid, often frightening dreams and can also get sleep paralysis.

The best-known symptom is the sudden loss of muscle control triggered by laughter, surprise, fear or anger. It can be anything from a slight feeling of weakness and limp muscles to sudden total body collapse, during which the person looks asleep, but is in fact awake and alert. The attacks last from a few seconds up to 30 minutes.

Scientists have found a chemical in the brain that patients with narcolepsy seem to lack. Also, their rapid eye movement (REM) sleep, which is when you're most likely to

Here's an idea for you

Write down the times when you're normally overcome with fatigue, so during these danger times you can make sure you're in a nap-friendly environment. As well as drug therapy, many experts recommend two or three short naps during the day to help control sleepiness and maintain alertness.

dream, seems to be all over the place. Normally, someone falls into REM sleep after about 90 minutes of sleep, but someone with narcolepsy can fall into REM sleep immediately so will often experience dreamlike imagery before the brain's asleep. REM episodes occur now and then in the day too – which is why people suffer hallucinations while they're awake.

Misdiagnosis as conditions such as depression and attention deficit disorder is common, and potentially dangerous since some treatments for these conditions can exacerbate narcolepsy.

Narcolepsy can't be cured, but with medication you'll be able to live a fairly normal life. Modafinil is most commonly prescribed for excessive daytime sleepiness, and Ritalin – known as the medication prescribed to children with attention deficit hyperactivity disorder (ADHD) when it is used to calm them down and help them focus on their tasks – helps to make people with narcolepsy more alert. Tricyclic antidepressants have been used to help improve muscle control and REM symptoms

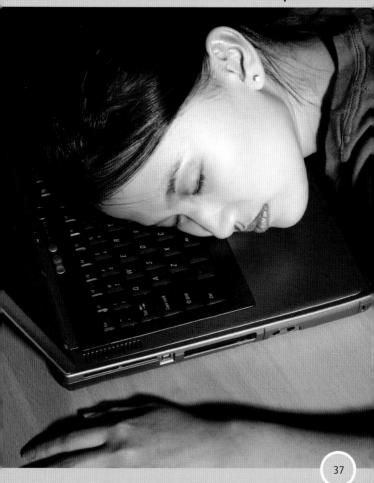

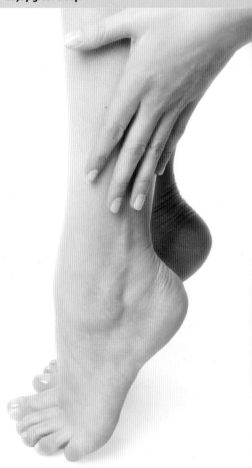

13. Itches and twitches

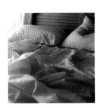

From tossing and turning to constant kicking, some people can't stop moving all night long

The main symptom of restless legs syndrome (RLS) is an unpleasant burning, prickling, tickling or aching feeling in your leg muscles, mainly in the calf, when you're inactive or relaxing. Some people also suffer involuntary jerking movements in their legs. Chances are, you are sleep deprived. You're probably taking more than half an hour to get to sleep and could be waking up three or more times in the night. It tends to run in families, is more common in women and the risk goes up as you get older. Pregnant women are also more prone.

Although its cause is unknown, RLS has been associated with other conditions, which if treated, can help. It can be a symptom of a deficiency in iron, vitamin B12 or folic acid; taking supplements will

Here's an idea for you

Track your progress. Keep a record of how any changes in lifestyle affect the symptoms of restless legs syndrome and the quality of your sleep. Every three days try something new so you can establish what makes a difference. Give each strategy a mark out of 10 where 1 is 'useless' and 10 is 'worked like a dream'.

normally sort it out. Nerve damage associated with rheumatoid arthritis, kidney failure or diabetes may also cause RLS – once the underlying condition is treated, RLS will probably get better. Certain medications including lithium, anticonvulsants, antidepressants and beta-blockers are also thought to be triggers – so changing to other drugs can help. Smoking, drinking alcohol and having too much caffeine seems to make RLS symptoms worse.

Irregular sleep habits may make you more tired and make RLS symptoms worse. If you've got RLS, you're more likely to sleep better later in the night – from about 2am to 10am. Good pre-bed rituals to try are pacing up and down, performing a stretching routine that includes leg work, taking a bath, massaging your legs with oil or applying hot or cold packs. A TENs machine strapped to your legs will emit vibrating electrical impulses which can block the aching and tickling sensations in your leg. If lifestyle changes don't work your doctor can tailor-make a drug-treatment programme for you.

14. What a grind!

When teeth grinding keeps you up at night

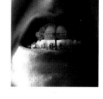

Teeth grinding or bruxism, is a condition where you either press, clench, or physically grind your teeth against each other. The most likely trigger is stress. You may wake up with a headache, jaw ache or earache that goes away as the day wears on. These are all are caused by joint and muscle strain in your upper and lower jaws. If left untreated, the surface of your upper and lower teeth can be worn down so much it creates an imbalance in closure between the left and right sides of your mouth. This can lead to gum disease and you may even lose some of your teeth. Your dentist will detect the characteristic wear on the teeth. Wear associated with grinding is most evident on the molars in the back of your mouth.

You need to tackle the cause and stop the situation getting any worse. Cut down on caffeine and alcohol, which make stress worse. Meditation and body-calming activities like yoga seem to help reduce the stress that aggravates habitual grinding. To relax

Here's an idea for you

Write down what sets off your teeth grinding in the day, then find an activity to do every time you feel the urge. This could be slow, deep breathing for instance. Place 'don't grind' reminders around the house on post-its. If you break the habit during the day this may help stop the grinding at night.

Defining idea

'Be true to your teeth and they won't
be false to you.'
SOUPY SALES, US TV presenter.

clenched muscles before you go to
bed or in the morning, apply a warm
face cloth to the side of your face.

Your dentist might recommend
muscle relaxants to relax your jaw
muscles or fit you with a special mouth guard for either jaw, to be worn
at night. This removable plastic device prevents teeth from coming
together, stopping further damage to your teeth and may also stop the
urge to grind. To treat the damage caused by more serious cases of
grinding, your dentist may reshape your biting surfaces with crowns or
inlays.

15. Ahhhhhhhh!!!

Scary monsters or your overbearing boss...don't let nightmares and night terrors ruin your sleep.

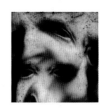

About 5–10 per cent of adults get nightmares once a month. You'll normally have your nightmare during the second half of the night in REM (dream) sleep. Suddenly you'll be woken up by a particularly harrowing episode. You'll be scared, anxious, very alert and will probably be able to recall your nightmare in great detail. Then you'll have trouble getting back to sleep.

Night terrors suddenly appear out of deep non-dreaming sleep and normally happen in the first half of the night. In a night terror, you'll sit up suddenly and scream – but you probably won't wake up even though your eyes might be wide open. You might sweat and your heart rate could shoot up to three times its normal rate – much higher than with nightmares. Amazingly, you'll probably have no

Here's an idea for you

If you have had a particular nightmare more than once, recall it in as much detail as you can, and write it down. Think about how you could change the outcome of the dream. Find 10–20 minutes of quiet and in a comfortable position, close your eyes, relax and visualise the new outcome of your dream. When the imagined dream has ended, write it down. The idea is that when you have the same dream again it will have your new ending.

43

Defining idea

'I don't use drugs, my dreams are frightening enough.'
M C ESCHER

memory of it in the morning, just a vague sense of frightening images.

After you've had a nightmare or night terror, write down any factors that may have contributed to the bad dream and see if you can deal with them. What did you eat yesterday? Fatty and spicy food as well as cheese are thought to increase the chance of nightmares. Did you have any alcohol or are you on medication? Are you stressed? Did you go to bed at a different time from usual? Did you watch a scary film? Are you ill?

The cause may not be obvious. With nightmares, talking through them – even drawing images from them – can help. With night terrors, talking often doesn't help because you can't remember the content. If they're really severe and happen often, talk to your doctor about medication.

16. Dreamworks

Control your dreams and tackle everyday problems.

With a bit of practice you can learn to use dreams to sort out problems. And this could mean you sleep better too.

You can easily get into the habit of interpreting your dreams and you may even be able to control them without the help of a therapist. Make a habit of remembering your dreams. Keep a dream journal handy by your bed and record every dream you remember, no matter how fragmentary. Write them all down, even if all you can recall is a face or a room. Remind yourself as you're falling asleep that you want to wake up fully from your dreams and remember them.

After a week, look back at your dream journal and try to work out what it means. Think about the

Here's an idea for you

Try this experiment to see if you can influence your dreams. Before you go to bed imagine dreaming about (1) finding a light switch, (2) turning it on, then turning it off, (3) turning on a light switch by willing it to happen and not touching the switch. Then see if any of these crop up in your dreams. In tests, 42 per cent of people were able to incorporate these three tasks in their dream.

Defining idea

*'A dream is a wish your heart makes,
when you're fast asleep.'*
Disney World advertisement

issues you have at work or in your relationship. Your dreams may point to problems you may not have thought of.

Learning to control your dreams – called lucid dreaming – is harder. This is when you realise you're dreaming, and then learn how to manipulate the dream. For example if you have an interview coming up, run through your mind the dialogue of the perfect interview. If you then dream about the interview going well, it will put you in the right frame of mind for the actual event. If you're trying to change the outcome of a recurrent dream or nightmare, when you're awake write out the script of how you'd like it to end. Then read and visualise it for 10 minutes before you go to bed.

17. On the move

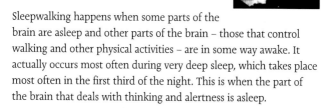

What should you do when there's a sleepwalker in the house?

Sleepwalking happens when some parts of the brain are asleep and other parts of the brain – those that control walking and other physical activities – are in some way awake. It actually occurs most often during very deep sleep, which takes place most often in the first third of the night. This is when the part of the brain that deals with thinking and alertness is asleep.

You're more likely to sleepwalk if you're sleep deprived as you fall into a deep sleep more quickly. Hormonal ups and downs in puberty, pregnancy and even menstruation increase the chances of sleepwalking. Stress is a trigger and drinking alcohol can also lead to sleepwalking.

Children are most likely to sleepwalk as they spend more of the night in deep sleep, when sleepwalking generally occurs. If your child sleepwalks, it's likely you

Here's an idea for you

If one of your family is sleepwalking, just gently guide them back to bed. Sleepwalkers who are suddenly woken up may be upset and have trouble falling asleep again. If the sleepwalker is in a dangerous situation, then you need to take some safety measures - particularly if the sleepwalker is a child. You should keep doors and windows closed and locked.

or a member of you family also did so when you were a child. The good news is that children tend to grow out of it. Adult sleepwalking is more serious as it's often more extreme, and so has more potential for self-injury. One study of adult sleepwalkers found that 19 per cent had been injured while sleepwalking.

If sleepwalking is getting you down, you need to tackle the cause. If it's triggered by alcohol, cut down and try not to drink after 10pm. If you're sleep deprived or stressed, deal with these, and the sleepwalking will probably stop. See your doctor about stress management techniques, counselling and relaxation exercises. The complementary therapies biofeedback, which teaches you to control various body functions, and hypnosis have been successful for sleepwalkers. As a last resort, talk to your doctor about drugs such as benzodiazepines, which can treat sleepwalking by relaxing your muscles and preventing movement.

18. Open all hours

Working the overnight shift? How to make sure you're getting enough sleep.

When you stay awake at night you're fighting your body clock, which is telling you to go to sleep. It's like getting jet lag every few days and can mean feeling groggy and tired all week. Many of the health and other problems associated with shift work are similar to those caused by sleep deprivation – higher risk of accidents and errors at work, increased chance of heart disease and poor concentration. So follow the tips below to minimise risk.

As far as you can, choose shifts that work with your body clock. If you're a night owl an evening and night shift would be best for you. If you're a lark, you'll be happy to start work at 6am, but would probably not be able to cope with a night shift. If you finish your shift in the day, wear wraparound sunglasses on the way home – exposure to bright light in the morning may reset your body clock and make it difficult to sleep.

Here's an idea for you

Unhappy with your work life balance? Work out if the advantages of your job are worth the trade off. Make a list of your values and priorities. Then cross off the items on your list that are not really all that important to you. Once you're down to two or three important values, you can see whether your lifestyle and your life fit with those values.

Defining idea

'Dawn: When men of reason go to bed'
AMBROSE BIERCE, US writer

At work, don't leave the boring stuff until the end of the day – you might find it difficult to finish. And if you're getting sleepy at the end of your shift, either go for a short break or ask one of your colleagues to step in for you. You will do the same for them.

Avoid heavy meals and alcohol before sleeping – they will make it harder to sleep. If you need to sleep during the day, make sure your home is sleep-friendly. Invest in heavy blinds to blackout the bedroom. Turn off the phone's ringer. Make sure your family knows not to interrupt you. Tell your neighbours about your shift work so they can keep the noise down in the day.

19. The jet set

Brilliant ways to beat jet lag

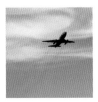

When you travel across time zones so fast that
your body doesn't have time to adjust to the new day and night
cues you mess with your internal body clock, causing symptoms
similar to those of a terrible hangover. Hopefully, these tips from
airline crews can soften the blow.

Work out the best time to travel to minimise the effects. An
overnight flight is best if you're travelling east, a day flight if going
west. If you're heading west, try to go to bed and get up an hour
later each day for a week before
your trip. If you're going east go to
bed earlier than usual.

Change your watch to your
destination time as soon as your
plane takes off. This will help get
your mind thinking in the new
time and help your body to adapt
itself to a different time zone.

Here's an idea for you

Apply a few drops of essential oil of
tangerine, bergamot or lemon to the
inside of your wrist or behind your ears
to pep you up once you've arrived. Or
unwind with lavender or clary sage after
a long flight.

Defining idea

'I love to travel but I hate to arrive'
ALBERT EINSTEIN

Try to sleep at the new times on the plane. If you need to keep yourself awake, do crossword puzzles or listen to stimulating music. Don't read a novel or watch the video – they're guaranteed to send you into a slumber. If you need to sleep, buy ear plugs.

During the flight, try to walk around as much as you can and, when sitting down, flex and extend your ankles to increase circulation. When you reach your destination, half an hour of exercise, such as a brisk walk, will keep you alert for up to two hours.

When you arrive in the new time zone, adjust your sleep schedule straight away to the local time. So if you arrive in the day but your body thinks it's night time, go outside, get lots of sunshine and keep active to trick your body into staying awake. Eat your meals at the local time, too. If you have to, take a 20 minute nap to help you get through the day.

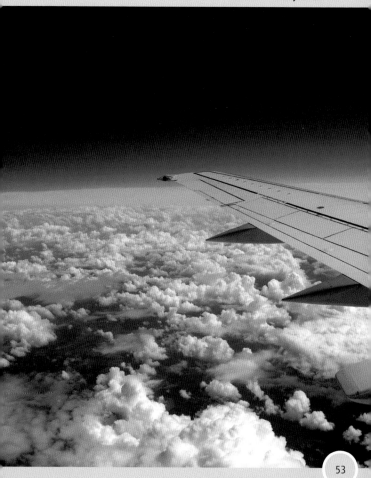

20. Dozy driving

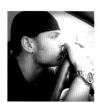

How to prevent falling asleep at the wheel

Tired drivers perform as poorly as drink drivers and studies show that drivers who have been awake for 15 hours or more are 4 times more likely to have an accident than a person who has had a good night's sleep. Ideally, you should only ever drive when well rested. In the real world, that's not always possible, so here are a few stay-awake strategies.

- Travel with another person. Chatting will help keep you alert. If you've got children in the car, play games such as I spy or First one to see....
- Between 12pm and 8am, and 1pm and 3pm are when you naturally feel most tired. If you must drive during these times, be extra vigilant.
- If you're on a long journey, schedule regular stops every 150 km or 2 hours. Stop sooner if tired.

Here's an idea for you

Stay alert with essential oils. Drop a few drops of stimulating oils such as lime, peppermint, lemongrass, black-pepper onto a tissue, then every time you need a boost take an energising sniff.

Defining idea

'The urge to continue driving despite acute feelings of sleepiness is rooted in a firm belief that "it won't happen to me'
PERETZ LAVIE, psychiatrist

- Okay I've said it's a no no, but if you're tired at the wheel, caffeine is a guaranteed way to pep you up. Feeling dehydrated can also make you tired – so drink plenty of water too.
- When you're tired, pull over to a rest area, roll up the windows, lock the doors, and lie back for about 15 minutes.
- Play music you love. Stay away from snooze-inducing sounds such as classical tracks and slow ballads. Go for loud, fast paced music that you can sing along to.
- Being hungry will make your blood sugar levels fall and make you even more tired. So keep handy some dried apricots, nuts, raisins or dried banana.

21. All stressed out!

Juggling work and home life? Busier than ever? No wonder your sleep is suffering.

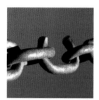

With expectations skyrocketing all the time –
we now want the perfect relationship, a beautiful home, model
children, a high performance car and wonderful holidays – it's no
surprise that stress levels are at an all time high as we fail to meet
these unachievable goals. It only needs a stressful life event such as a
divorce or death, moving home or a new job to tip you over the edge.

A certain amount of stress is good for us – it makes us perform
better. In the past a shot of adrenaline and cortisol would pump us
up for fighting enemies or running
away from danger. The problem
today is that instead of just using
these stress hormones in
emergencies, we are now living at
such a pace that we activate them
all the time – like when we're
going to miss a train, or when
someone records over our favourite
video tape. The result? Sleep
problems...

Here's an idea for you

Start a stress diary. For at least two
weeks, keep a list of events, times,
places and people that seem to make
you feel more stressed. You'll probably
be surprised to find that a pattern soon
emerges. Once you've identified your
pressure points you can work out how
to deal with them.

Defining idea

'A ruffled mind makes a restless pillow'
CHARLOTTE BRONTE

Stress not only makes it more difficult to sleep because the stress hormones are keeping your mind active, it also depletes the sleep hormones serotonin and melatonin so you can't relax. On top of this, stress reduces the amount of deep sleep you get, making the sleep you do get lighter and less satisfactory. And you're more likely to wake up in the middle of the night. Then, of course, you get anxiety dreams – who hasn't suffered the humiliation of walking through their office with no clothes on? Fortunately, however, for most people, sleep returns to normal when the factor causing the stress is removed.

22. Say no to stress

Calm-down strategies to stop night-time niggles

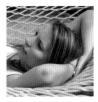

Once you've worked out which people and events trigger your stress, talk through it with a good friend or your partner – even the act of discussing things often makes you feel better. Ask for impartial advice on easing the problems that you've discovered. Once you know your stress triggers, try to nip them in the bud. Changing your routine can help as can practising a few relaxation or breathing exercises as soon as your stress levels start to rise.

There's nothing more stressful than being disorganised, so get your life in order. If you've got a list of jobs that need doing, set yourself two tasks and make sure you do them. Then whatever else the day throws at you, at least you'll have achieved something. Research shows that people who patiently complete one task at a time, with undivided attention have more calm energy than those who try to do too many

Here's an idea for you

To banish stress related headaches and insomnia, try hand reflexology. Stretch out your right hand and, with your left thumb, apply pressure from the base of your hand, working your way up to the top of your thumb tip. Repeat ten times.

Defining idea

'For fast-acting relief, try slowing down'
LILY TOMLIN, actress and comedian

things at once. Juggling projects increase tension, which lowers energy. So allow yourself plenty of time to complete a task.
If you tackle the worst task first everything else will seem easier.

Plan breaks in your day. Get up 15 minutes earlier than you think you need to and prepare for the day without rushing. You'll leave the house in a calmer, more positive mood. And try to have 20 minutes in the morning and afternoon that is exclusively 'your' time, in which you can do whatever you want, even if it is simply sitting doing nothing.

Finally, don't let a work problem such as bullying get out of control. Keep a record of all the incidents, including copies of all letters and emails written by the bully, and record all criticisms in writing. Then you'll be fully armed to take up the matter with management.

23. Sunday night insomnia

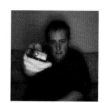

**Make sure Monday morning doesn't ruin
Sunday night by following the tips below.**

■ Don't lie in at the weekend, this is one of the reasons you feel more tired on a Monday morning. Every time you sleep in you delay the rise in your body temperature, which means you delay the time you're likely to get to sleep the following night.

■ Select a time every weekend when you deal with the troublesome thoughts that normally keep you awake on Sunday night. Write down all the things worrying you and come up with ways to tackle them. You should find it easier to sleep knowing that you have a strategy and that you're in control of the situation.

■ Eating a huge meal at Sunday lunch time will make you feel sluggish and desperate for an afternoon snooze. But if you do take a nap you'll find it harder to sleep that night, giving you a bad start to the week. Eat a light meal and go for a stroll an hour after eating to ward off lethargy.

Here's an idea for you

Save time and cut morning stress by preparing for work the night before. So wash and blow-dry your hair and lay out a clean, ironed outfit for the next day. If you've got children, lay out their clothes and bags.

Defining idea

'It is better to sleep on things beforehand than lie awake about them afterward'

BALTASAR GRACIAN, Spanish philosopher

- One way of tackling Sunday insomnia is to use Sunday evening to plan a treat for Monday or Tuesday. This could be a meal out, going to the cinema or getting together with friends. Focusing on something positive will stop you dreading the following Monday morning.

- Practise moderate drinking. If you regularly have more than the recommended amount of alcohol at weekends (over three units a day for women or four for men) you'll sleep less well at the weekend making Monday morning more of a struggle.

- Don't bring work home at the weekend – it's guaranteed to make you feel as if you haven't had a break when you get back to work on Monday morning. Talk to your boss about how you can plan your time more efficiently or delegate some of your workload.

24. More than just the blues

When depression saps your sleep time

Most people feel down now and again – it's only a problem if it doesn't go away and your sleep is still suffering. Depression is often triggered by stress, bereavement, financial problems or difficult relationships and having a negative outlook makes you more prone as it makes you less able to cope. As a result, there'll be a drop in the key chemicals in your brain responsible for regulating mood – serotonin and noradrenaline. You need serotonin to produce your sleep-inducing melatonin, so it's inevitable your sleep will suffer.

Your doctor will give you an assessment to make sure you haven't got another underlying condition such as an underactive thyroid or anaemia which can also make you tired. He may prescribe antidepressants which affect the levels of your brain chemicals. Selective serotonin reuptake inhibitors (SSRIs) like Prozac work by

Here's an idea for you

Dwelling on past hurts will make you feel bitter and resentful, so savour your positive past and plan your future. Every day for a whole week, set aside five minutes each morning and night to think about some of the loveliest things you've experienced. Take a pen and paper and imagine who and where you want to be, then work out what steps you need to take.

Defining idea

'Noble deeds and hot baths are the best cures for depression'
DODIE SMITH, English author

boosting serotonin levels. Others such as amitriptylines, act as a sedative as well as increasing serotonin. The most effective treatment, however, is some form of talking therapy on its own or combined with medication.

Once you've discovered why you're depressed and learned how to cope, your depression is less likely to come back. Psychoanalysts often blame depression on an inability to deal with anger and a desperate need for approval. You'll have to delve deep into the past to resolve these issues and this can take years. Cognitive therapists believe depressed people are caught in a cycle of negative thinking and expect to fail. Your therapist will help change the way you think. Counselling can be useful if your depression is triggered by one specific problem.

25. Baby on the way

As a rule, most symptoms get worse as your bump gets bigger. Oh the joys of pregnancy...

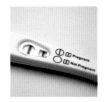

0–3 months Rising levels of the hormone progesterone may make you feel drowsy in the day but disrupt your sleep at night, leading to even more fatigue during the next morning. Nausea could also keep you awake. The most common reason for disrupted sleep, however, is going to the toilet.

3–6 months You might find you're more tired, but spend most of the time in bed tossing and turning, trying to find a comfortable position. At its most extreme this turns into restless legs syndrome. You may suffer cramps in your calves as your leg muscles struggle to cope with the extra weight. You could start to get heartburn at night, triggered by the growing uterus putting extra pressure on your stomach.

6–9 months You may develop nasal congestion, causing you to snore. Also prepare for severe back pains that interfere with your sleep. Nightmares are more common.

Here's an idea for you

Still uncomfortable? Lie on your side with your knees bent and a pillow between your knees. Arrange other pillows under your belly and behind your back for extra support.

Towards the end of pregnancy, the discomfort and movement of your baby could mean you're awake nearly all night.

- Avoid drinking for an hour or two before bed to limit night-time trips to the toilet.
- Eat a light, high-carbohydrate snack before you go to bed to keep nausea at bay.
- Avoid heartburn by eating small, frequent meals rather than three large ones. Lay off citrus, spices, fried foods, and chocolate because they can irritate the oesophagus. Sit up after eating. Sleeping on several pillows might help.
- Train yourself to sleep on your side. Sleeping flat on your back can restrict breathing and may reduce blood flow to the baby if the uterus presses on the main artery of your body, the aorta.
- If you have restless legs syndrome (RLS), you may have been deficient in iron or folic acid before becoming pregnant – your doctor may prescribe vitamin supplements.
- To stop cramps, try stretching your calf by flexing your foot, heel first, gently massaging your leg, placing a hot water bottle on the cramped area, or getting up and walking around.

26. Cry babies

Sleep deprivation caused by babies and young children.

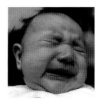

Sometimes children wake up because as babies they never learned how to fall asleep on their own. Babies can become dependant on being held, sung to, rocked, breastfed, given a bottle, or even driven in a car in order to fall asleep.

If you always hold or rock your baby until he is completely asleep, rather than putting him down in the crib when he is drowsy but still a little bit awake, your baby develops a habit of having to be in your arms before he can fall asleep. Your baby associates the feeling of being held with the process of falling to sleep. Without the holding, he simply can't fall asleep. And if you give your baby a bottle to fall asleep with, he may come to rely on that as a trigger for sleep. Soon you'll find yourself fixing bottles two or three times a night.

An illness can also set you back. Your child may have been sleeping through the night for months, but then get an ear infection, a cold or start teething. Your child may get

Here's an idea for you

By three or four months, make it a habit to put your baby down to sleep when she's drowsy but not yet fully asleep. That way, she won't develop a habit of having to be held by you each time she wakes in the middle of the night.

Defining idea

'People who say they sleep like a baby usually don't have one'
REVEREND LEO J. BURKE

used to being comforted at night so once the pain has gone he may whimper in the hope of some attention. Can you blame him?

If you don't deal with nighttime wakings, the problem probably won't go away. Soon your child will start coming into your bed and before you know it, the family is playing musical beds. I know plenty of families where the dad either ends up on his own under his daughter's Barbie duvet cover or downstairs on the sofa, while mum is sandwiched between two fidgety young children.

27. No baby no cry

The plan that stops your kids waking you up at night

The key to every child's sleeping habits is the right bedtime routine. Once you've worked out a schedule, stick to it and keep bed times and waking times consistent seven days a week. Having daytime routines such as regular meal and activity times also helps anchor sleep times.

Most cases of night time waking can be cured easily by controlled crying where you teach your child to go to sleep on her own. If you're really tough, you can probably solve it in two or three nights by letting her cry and not going to her at all. In theory, she'll cry for 20 or 30 minutes the first night, 10 minutes the second night, not at all the third.

If you find this approach too harsh sit down by your baby's cot without turning on the light and keep murmuring something reassuring such as, 'Don't worry, mummy (or daddy) is here. Go back to sleep' until she does. Do

Here's an idea for you

Try writing out your child's bed time rituals like a script in order to make it consistent and put it up on the kitchen notice board where everyone can see it. They should be simple so that grandma or your babysitter can follow them if you're not around.

Defining idea

'Too many parents make life hard for
their children by trying, too zealously,
to make it easy for them'
GOETHE

less and less every night to comfort
your baby until she's going to sleep
on her own. If the first night you
lightly stroke your baby, on the
second night continue the
soothing voice but don't stroke
your child. This approach does
take longer.

A compromise solution involves letting your child cry for two
minutes on the first night, then going in and reassuring her briefly,
tucking her in and leaving. On subsequent nights let her cry for five,
then ten, then fifteen minutes and so on before going in to comfort
her and leaving. This usually works in a few nights, but may take up
more of your night, so do it at a weekend when you and your
partner can do shifts and make up for lost sleep the next day.

28. Change those sheets!

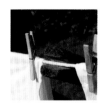

Does your child wet the bed? Here's how to sort it out and restore your night's sleep.

Most children who wet the bed seem to be very deep sleepers. Whereas other children wake up when they sense that their bladders are full, your child may simply have difficulty rousing. And some kids just need to wee more at night – maybe due to a smaller-than-average bladder.

If your child isn't ready to sleep without night nappies, don't force him. All of you will sleep better if your child stays in nappies at night until he's ready to stay dry. If he sometimes wakes up dry or his nappy is barely damp in the morning, he may be ready to try, but be prepared to go back to nappies if this doesn't work. Tell him in a reassuring way that his body isn't ready to stay dry at night yet, and try again in a few months.

Here's an idea for you

Get your child to take responsibility by helping to change the sheets. This is not a punishment. The idea is that children will often feel better by helping with the cleaning-up process.

Defining idea

'All kids need is a little help, a little hope and somebody who believes in them.'
EARVIN 'MAGIC' JOHNSON

Your child's bedwetting will probably resolve itself naturally – with the right encouragement, support and positive reinforcement. Offering incentives like a small treat if they wake up dry can work. Whatever you do, don't punish your child for bedwetting. This will make him feel bad and will probably make the problem worse. No one wets the bed on purpose.

Reassure him that it's a common problem and explain the condition – buy a book about bedwetting aimed at children. The more they know about the condition, the more likely it is they'll be able to overcome it.

If your child is over six, he could try a buzzer alarm – a device which wakes him when he wets. This eventually teaches him to wake when he needs to go. You may need to get your doctor to refer you to a sleep expert, however, to learn how to use it properly.

29. Forget the lie in!

Coping with children who wake up too early

If your child is waking up before getting a full night's sleep, check to see whether something in her bedroom is rousing him or keeping her awake. If sunlight is streaming through the window at the crack of dawn, for instance, hang curtains lined with blackout fabric or add a room darkening shade or blind. The light is normally what tells the brain to wake up – but some children are more sensitive to it than others.

If your child is sleepy and wants to take a nap soon after rising – particularly if she's past the daytime napping stage – she's probably not getting enough sleep at night. If she wakes early in the morning and you think she needs more rest, encourage her to go back to sleep. If your child is still in a cot then instead of rushing into her room the moment you hear a peep, wait ten or 15 minutes – even if she's crying. She may just turn over and go back to sleep.

Here's an idea for you

Start a star chart. Give your child a star every time she stays in her room until an agreed time – say, 7 o'clock. After 10 stars, allow her to choose a small treat from your local toy shop. If you're lucky – just getting the stars will be incentive enough.

73

Defining idea

'What is a home without children? Quiet.'
HENNY YOUNGMAN, comedian

Your toddler can sleep only so much. For some children, a later bedtime will help. If your child's going to bed at 7, try tucking her in about ten minutes later every night until 7.30 or 8. But if you want a lie in, don't be tempted to put her to bed really late. Overtired children rarely sleep well and she'll probably get up the same time as she usually does and just be grumpy the next day.

Encourage your child to play in her cot with a favourite toy for a few minutes. If your child's older, try to get her to play with the toys in your bedroom until an agreed time – say, 7 o'clock. She doesn't need to be able to tell the time – just recognise when the big hand's at the 12 and the little hand's at the 7.

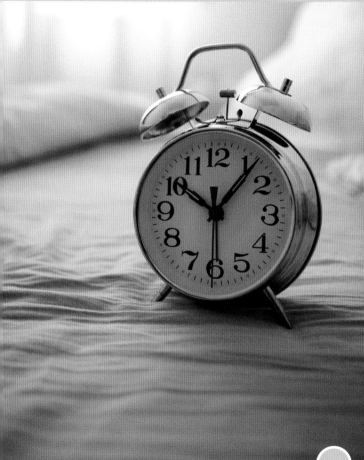

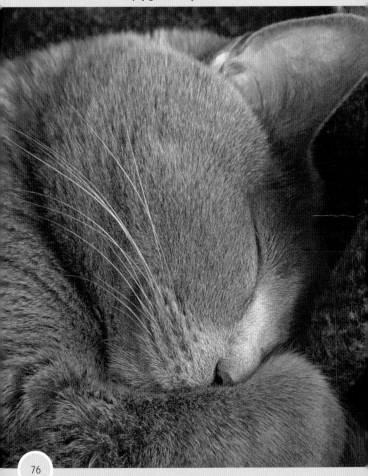

30. Forty winks

Does the power nap really work?

We're designed for two sleeps a day – the main one at night and a nap in the afternoon. If you're getting enough sleep at night, you'll probably be okay – a handful of nuts may be all you need to pep you up. If you're sleep deprived, though, you could be under par all afternoon. According to fans of napping, a 15- to 20-minute nap can restore alertness and memory and relieve stress and fatigue.

In reality, though, it's often difficult to nap, but even if you don't actually fall asleep, 20 minutes of quiet time may give you the boost you need.

- Find somewhere quiet such as an empty office and turn off the phone.
- Loosen your clothing and take off your shoes. Lie down on a sofa, stretch out on the floor or if that's not possible sit comfortably on a chair, placing your head in your folded arms on your desk.

Here's an idea for you

To discover how naps affect your energy level and the quality of your nighttime sleep, do an experiment. Take a daily nap for a week. The next week, don't nap. Every morning, rank your sleep quality on a 10-point scale. Every evening, rate your day on a similar scale. After two weeks, judge whether naps work for you.

Defining idea

'No day is so bad it can't be fixed with
a nap'
CARRIE SNOW, comedian

- Close your eyes – ideally, put on an eye mask and try not to think about work or all the things you have to do. Focus on what you love doing in your spare time.

- Don't try to sleep – if your brain needs a rest, you'll soon fall asleep.

- If you do nap, set an alarm clock to wake you 15–20 minutes later. Don't sleep for more than 30 minutes – you'll wake up groggier and foggier.

- When you wake up lie still for a minute or two – then stretch and breathe deeply and take a drink of water or a light snack to get your system going again.

- Return to work, starting with simple chores such as opening letters or organising the work you have to do. Within just a few minutes you should feel sparky again.

31. Pill popping

The lowdown on sleeping pills: are they really a short cut to good sleep?

Sleeping pills can be a good short term measure. However, you can get physically – as well as psychologically – addicted to sleeping pills. You take them every day and get a good night's sleep, but as soon as you stop taking them the sleeplessness returns. Why? You haven't dealt with what's causing your insomnia and you still can't go to sleep on your own. Many doctors prefer giving out anti-depressants which they think is a lower risk option and helps tackle the cause of insomnia.

Sleeping pills work by depressing your brain activity and slowing down brainwaves. They also relieve anxiety symptoms and relax your muscles. The difference between the various brands is usually the time it takes to break them down and get them out of your system. This can be anything from a few hours to days – the longer they

Here's an idea for you

To ensure you get the right pill for you, describe your problem to your doctor precisely – whether you can't go to sleep or you wake up frequently, whether you're stressed or depressed, for instance. Make sure they explain how the drug prescribed works, the possible side effects, and how long it's likely to be effective. Insist on the lowest dose pack. You don't want to get hooked on a higher dose that at some time you will need to wean yourself off.

Defining idea

'Reality is just a crutch for people who can't cope with drugs'
ROBIN WILLIAMS

hang around, the more likely you are to feel drowsy or suffer other side effects. The longer you use sleeping pills, the more your brain gets used to them and the less effective they are. Of course, the answer is *not* to increase your dose but to stop taking them.

There are two types of sleeping pills most commonly prescribed – benzodiazepines such as temazepam, flurazepam and lorazepam which help relax muscles and imidazopyridines and cyclopyrrolones such as zolpidem, salepon and zoplicone which also relax the muscles. They don't last as long as the first type but they're less addictive and you're less likely to feel drowsy in the day. You may have to try a few before you find one that suits you.

32. Mind power

With a bit of direction, you can reign in your thoughts and think yourself sleepy. Here's how...

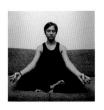

First off, you probably need to become more positive about sleep – particularly if you've got to the stage that you dread going to bed, convinced that you're never going to get a good night's sleep again. This mindset will make your insomnia worse. Try to replace any negative thoughts with positive but realistic ones such as, 'As long as I get some sleep and relax my body, I'll be fine.' Writing down your affirmation may speed up the process of believing the affirmation.

Good sleepers cultivate strong mental associations of physical relaxation, mental calm, and good sleep with their bedtime, their bed and bedroom, and their bedtime rituals like brushing their teeth and setting the alarm clock. Learn to become a good sleeper by making these same associations. Practicing muscle relaxation while you're brushing your teeth and deep breathing while you're

Here's an idea for you

Can't visualise a peaceful or relaxing scene? Why not think of a situation or place that you've always found really boring. Recapture that bored, tired, heavy, sleepy feeling that you always experience. Let that feeling spread through your mind and all through your body until you're overcome with tiredness.

Defining idea

'I really can't be expected to drop everything and start counting sheep at my age. I hate sheep'
DOROTHY PARKER

putting on your pyjamas. Imagine your bed is a huge white fluffy cloud and that all your worries disappear the moment you step into it.

Take this visualisation further when you're in bed by conjuring up an image of something relaxing. Just lie there with your eyes closed and imagine you're in your favourite, most peaceful place. Try to experience it in your head – see your surroundings, hear the peaceful sounds. Just relax and enjoy it – and drift off to sleep. Once you've found a place that's especially peaceful and effective, you'll find that the more you use it, the more you can count on it to help you relax and get to sleep.

33. Food for thought

What and when you eat affects how you sleep – so read on for the dinners to make you doze.

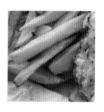

Eating healthily and regularly is one of the best ways to keep your energy levels high, preventing you from dropping off inappropriately in the day and ensuring your body releases all the hormones you need to send you off to sleep at night. The most effective sleep diet is to eat little and often keeping your metabolic rate steady. Meals that are high in carbohydrates and low-to-medium in protein will help you relax in the evening and set you up for a good night's sleep.

Your sleep can be affected by foods which take a long time to digest – high fat and high protein foods take twice as long as carbohydrate to metabolise. Avoid foods that perk you up and opt for ones that encourage restful sleep. Steer clear of foods containing the amino acid tyrosine – found in bacon, cured meat, strong cheese and chocolate – which stimulates the brain. Instead go for those containing

Here's an idea for you

Write down what and when you eat and drink in your sleep diary for a week and see if there's any link between your diet and how well you sleep. You can then start by avoiding any food that's causing problems.

Defining idea

'A light supper, a good night's sleep, and a fine morning have often made a hero of the same man who by indigestion, a restless night, and a rainy morning, would have proved a coward.'
LORD CHESTERFIELD

tryptophan – an amino acid that your body gets from certain foods and uses to make serotonin, which it then turns into sleep-inducing melatonin. Cottage cheese, milk, chicken, turkey, rice, eggs, beans, spinach and seafood all contain good amounts. To get the full snoozy effect, eat these foods with carbohydrates such as pasta or potatoes. After eating carbs, your body releases insulin, which helps clear the bloodstream of other amino acids that compete with tryptophan, meaning more tryptophan gets to the brain.

Key sleepy vitamins and minerals are vitamin B6, found in whole grains, bananas, dried apricots and potatoes; vitamin B3, found in red meat, chicken, oily fish and mushrooms; magnesium, in avocados, green leafy vegetables and nuts; and calcium from dairy products, broccoli and almonds.

34. Sleepy snacks

A bedtime snack can not only help you drop off, it can stop you waking up in the middle of the night with a rumbling tummy.

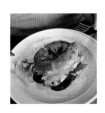

If you fall asleep easily but wake several hours later, it may be due to low blood sugar – and a light bite before bed could nip that in the bud. You need something that's high in complex carbohydrates, with a small amount of protein which contains just enough tryptophan to relax the brain. A bit of calcium on top of this works a treat – it helps the brain use the tryptophan to make sleep hormone melatonin. A bowl of porridge is probably the best sleep-inducing food of all as it contains complex carbohydrates, calcium and tryptophan. Some 40 minutes after eating it your levels of melatonin will rise, setting you up for a deep, restorative sleep.

Avoid all-carbohydrate snacks, especially those high in junk sugars like biscuits – they're less likely to

Here's an idea for you

Instead of hot milk, make this oaty alternative. Soak a level tablespoon of oatmeal in a little milk for an hour or so in a small saucepan. Add a large glass of milk and bring to the boil gently, stirring all the time until it has slightly thickened. Pour it back into a glass, then add a spoonful of honey and plenty of grated nutmeg. Drink, and you'll soon feel your eyelids get heavier and heavier...

help you sleep. You'll miss out on the sleep-inducing effects of tryptophan, and you may set off the roller-coaster effect of plummeting blood sugar followed by the release of stress hormones that will keep you awake.

Try one of these healthy snacks about 40 minutes before you settle down under your duvet. This gives them enough time to perform their magic...

■ Honey with oatcakes;
■ Wholemeal toast with cottage cheese and pineapple;
■ Bagel with low fat cream cheese and chopped dates;
■ Crackers and hummus;
■ Whole-grain cereal with milk;
■ Peanut butter sandwich with ground sesame seeds – both of which contain tryptophan.

35. Fit for sleep

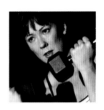

Did you know that regular exercise can actually help you drop off more quickly and sleep more soundly.

You need to do at least three hours of exercise per week to make a difference. Ten minutes three times a day works just as well as one half hour session. Although aerobic exercise – anything that gets your heart pumping faster – works best, lifting weights and stretching can also help your sleep.

The ideal time to exercise is late afternoon or evening – if you do a strenuous workout too close to bedtime your temperature may be still be too high for sleep.

■ Do something you enjoy – you'll only give up otherwise. If you're competitive, try team sports. If you're sociable, do a dance class or join a hiking club. If you need a challenge, try wall climbing or a martial art where you're learning a skill as well as getting fit.

Here's an idea for you

Start an exercise diary. Note down every activity you do every day and how long you did it for – even small things like walking to the bus stop. Then note how well you slept that night. Work out if any particular activity is helping you sleep. Once you've reached your weekly three-hour aerobic target, give yourself a reward.

Defining idea

'Whenever I feel like exercising, I lie down until the feeling passes.'
ROBERT MAYNARD HUTCHINS, education reformer

- Set a goal, such as swimming twenty lengths, as soon as you've reached your goal, set another.
- Change your activities regularly and do something you've never done before. Boredom is one of the main reasons people stop exercising.
- If you work regular hours, walk or cycle part or all of the way to work. Start with just once a week, then progress to two to three times a week.
- Make life a bit difficult for yourself. During your lunch hour, find a sandwich shop 15 minutes walk away rather than the one next to your office – and walk briskly. Use stairs rather than lifts or escalators.
- Keep giving up on your exercise video? Get a fan – a cool breeze will make you more alert and willing to hang on to the end.

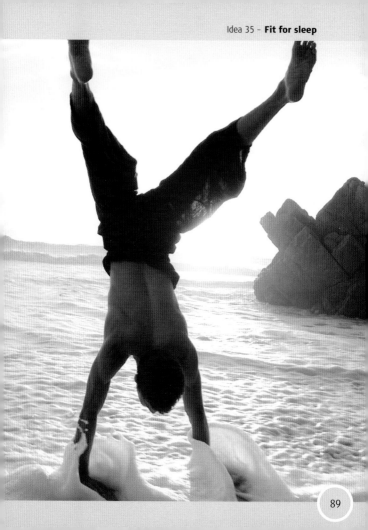

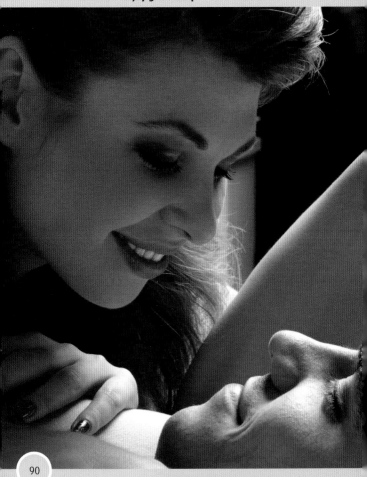

36. Sexual healing

Pep up your sex life – the most enjoyable way to beat insomnia.

When you have an orgasm, your body releases five times the normal level of the cuddle hormone oxytocin, which calms you down for sleep. Orgasms also produce a rush of endorphins which lift your spirits. And if headaches are preventing you from getting to sleep, sex may be just what the doctor ordered. Most headaches are tension headaches and muscle tension is usually found in your head, shoulders, neck or back. After you've had sex, the feel-good endorphins released act like a mild painkiller.

Most important, a good sex life brings you closer to your partner because of the intimacy you share. And if you're happy with your partner, it's one thing less to worry about when you're trying to get to sleep.

Here's an idea for you

Improve your orgasms – perform kegel exercises. By exercising the muscles you use to control your urine flow you can improve your control and your sensation during sex. Both men and women can do this. Just tense then relax these muscles slowly. Start by doing 10, building up to 100 a day.

Defining idea

'When I'm good I'm very, very good but when I'm bad I'm better.'
MAE WEST

Try these tips to rev up your sex life:

- Flirt with each other – over breakfast, while you're brushing your teeth, in the queue at the post office, everywhere.
- Throw your TV out of the bedroom – watching TV in bed kills off your sex life.
- Don't skip the kissing. It makes sex last longer and strengthens affection and arousal.
- Give each other a massage using sensual oils. For something a bit naughtier, try a body-to-body massage – man on his front, woman on top. Rub your body up and down his.
- Eat a banana in bed. A rich source of vitamin B, they enhance sex and orgasm by promoting the flow of blood to your sex organs.
- Go to bed naked – there's nothing like baggy jogging pants and a holey t-shirt to put you off sex. Leave a t-shirt by the bed if you get cold later.
- Talk to each other – it's the key to a good sex life and lively libido. Set aside half an hour each day just to catch up and talk.

37. Mattress matters

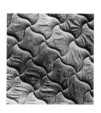

Is your bed soft or lumpy? Have you had it for more than 15 years? It may be time to look for a new one.

To relieve and prevent back pain you need a bed with the correct support and comfort. The idea is to keep your spine in correct alignment, while the bed moulds itself to your natural body contours. This will also mean you'll be moving around less. Remember, you're going to spend over 29,000 hours on your bed during an average lifespan so it's worth taking a little time and effort to make the right choice. Before you buy:

- Consider a bigger bed. Studies have shown that couples sleep better in a bigger bed – on average we prod each other 120 times a night.

- Look for a supportive rather than a hard bed. Correct support (which is dependent on your weight and build) coupled with comfort is best.

- Look at pocket sprung beds – they tend to feel softer, as they are packed with more

Here's an idea for you

Go into a shop with a list of your priorities and concerns in advance. There are so many different types of bed that you could be tempted by something you don't really need. Narrow your choice down to two or three and then spend plenty of time lying on these in your normal sleeping positions. Five or 10 minutes should be the minimum for each bed.

upholstery and also feature smaller, lighter springs than a conventional mattress. The springs are packed tightly together so they give good individual support.

■ Consider a waterbed. Lying on a waterbed is like floating and you get a feeling of weightlessness. The bed has a heater, so you can choose a temperature to suit you. Waterbeds also conform perfectly to your body, so you're less likely to move around.

■ Get a space bed – a foam mattresses based on NASA technology. The mattress stops tossing and turning by moulding to the shape and position of your body. When your spine is supported in the correct anatomical shape, there's less tossing and turning.

38. Snoozy rooms

Make your bedroom a sleep sanctuary.

If you dread going to bed because you have
too much to do or have difficulty falling asleep, try making bedtime
seem more luxurious so you'll look forward to it. For example,
invest in cotton sheets with a high thread count (at least 200 threads
per inch); they cost more but feel softer. Change your bedding about
once a week, or often enough to keep it feeling fresh. Subtly
scenting your bedroom with fragrant herbs can also make bedtime
feel special. Try stuffing a couple of tablespoons of dried lavender in
a small cloth bag and tucking it among your pillows. This acts as a
mild sedative, too.

Your bedroom environment should
calm you. That means no computers,
CD players, and television or piles of
books, magazines, letters, bills, and
dirty clothes, which can all make you
feel anxious and keep you awake. If
you must keep electronics in your
bedroom, at least turn them off

Here's an idea for you

Take an inventory of everything in your
bedroom then give it marks out of ten
according to how stimulating it is and
whether you think it stops you from
going to sleep. You should remove from
your bedroom everything that scores
over 5 out of 10.

95

Defining idea

'For sleep, one needs endless depths of blackness to sink into; daylight is too shallow, it will not cover one'
ANNE MORROW LINDBERGH, author

before bedtime and keep them out of your line of sight. Pictures are distracting too since they remain in your mind even after you've turned out the lights.

The darker it is when you sleep, the better your melatonin production, and the better the quality of your sleep. To block out light from outside always draw your blinds or curtains – and ideally invest in blackout versions which let in virtually no light. Turn brightly lit digital clocks around so you can't see them.

A slightly cool room contributes to good sleep – about 60-65°F (16–18°C). That's because it matches what occurs deep inside the body, when the body's internal temperature drops during the night to its lowest level.

39. What a racket!

Whether you're being kept awake by noisy neighbours or people playing loud music in their cars outside, think about noise proofing your bedroom.

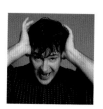

Timber floorboards make noise reverberate around the room – so consider fitting carpets or thick rugs to stop this. Close windows and doors when you want peace and quiet. Heavy curtains will help keep noise out.

Windows are the most common way for noise to get in. Single glass panes and wood window frames are the least resistant to noise. Fitting your window frames with thicker glass can help – twice as thick and your traffic noise will drop by half. Double glazing can reduce noise by about 20 per cent, while vinyl frames can reduce it by 50 per cent. A board or 'plug' made from special soundproofing material which you place over your window before you

Here's an idea for you

Test how well soundproofed your windows are. Seal gaps with plasticine, which can be removed without damaging paint surfaces. Test over several days and nights. If noise levels go down, think about fitting sealing devices on your windows which allow your windows to be opened, while maximising noise reduction when they're closed.

Defining idea

'He who sleeps in continual noise is wakened by silence'
WILLIAM DEAN HOWELLS,
American novelist

go to bed will block out both noise and light. The extra insulation of a plug will also keep you warmer in winter and cooler in summer.

As well as reducing your central heating bill, insulating your bedroom wall will reduce the amount of noise that's let in. If you're trying to block out the noise coming from your street, you only really need to soundproof that wall. The best way to do this is by dry lining, where the wall is lined with insulating material and covered in plasterboard.

Many attics, especially in older homes, have no insulation. Putting it in not only cuts down on your heating bills, it can help to soundproof your home. Extra layers of tarmac can also increase your home's noise tolerance, especially to aircraft. If you live near an airport, try stapling extra tarmac sheets on the roof rafters inside the attic – it's a cheap and effective way to reduce noise.

40. The Feng Shui bedroom

Feng Shui may sound like nonsense but if your sleep's suffering what harm can it do to try?

The idea behind Feng Shui is to increase harmony in your environment through maintaining good flow of chi, the invisible life force in everything around us. A disturbance in the flow of chi can ruin your sleep, relationships and health so check out the tips below.

If you have a choice of rooms, go for one that's towards the back of your house. Remove any clutter, especially under the bed – this is meant to indicate there's clutter in your relationship. Any furniture should be comfortable and safe with rounded or soft edges and corners.

Put the head of your bed against a solid wall so that when you're in it you feel safe and secure. Never put your bed under a window – this may lead to a lack of support from those

Here's an idea for you

If you really want to use white paint in your bedroom but are worried about draining the room's energy, you can always add splashes of bright red. The Chinese believe that red brings luck and red is used for healing, wealth, strength and vitality. Red curtains, a red throw or red cushions on your bed will boost the energy in your room.

around you. The rush of chi from the window could also cause restless sleep. Apparently, sleeping under a beam causes ill health, bad luck and relationship problems. Lastly, do not place your bed with the head or foot pointed at a door. This is known as the coffin position, and it drains away all your good luck and energy. Positioning your bed within sight of the door but off to one side promotes restful sleep.

Pairs of candlesticks, vases or picture frames are thought to increase marital harmony. Putting nightstands and lights on both sides of the bed invites your partner into your nest. If you want to hang pictures, opt for landscape posters of warm sunsets or grassy fields. Mirrors and anything that reflects or shines light are meant to bounce energy into different directions.

Adding colour to a room is a great way to get rid of bad energy. White is associated with death and mourning and drains energy, so pick colours like cream or antique white if you want a neutral colour.

41. Music to my ears

From whale music to Mozart, how to turn on, tune in, drop off...

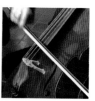

The right track can slow your breathing and your heart rate, relax your muscles and put you in a great mood. Most say that music to relax you before bed should be quiet, melodic with a slow beat and few, if any rhythmic accents. Listening to Pachelbel's Canon in D, for instance, at around 64 beats per minute, the rate of a resting heart beat, will slow your breathing rate and heart rate and change your brain wave pattern from rapid beta waves to the slower, sleepier alpha ones.

Find three songs that sound like you feel when you're stressed or down, three that sound like you want to feel when you're relaxed and three in between. Make a CD or put them on your MP3 player. The music should gradually become calmer, quieter and slower. Put this on in the evening and it will guide you through your feelings and lift your mood.

There are hundreds of relaxation CDs on the market – some simply for relaxing, some to beat insomnia and stress. If you don't fancy music, look to nature – you can now get

Here's an idea for you

Find out how music affects your heart rate. Listen to various pieces of music, fast and slow, and then take your pulse. Your heart will speed up or slow down to match the rhythm of a sound so if you're listening to a slower piece, your heart will beat slower to match it.

Defining idea

'Why waste money on psychotherapy when you can listen to the B Minor Mass?'
MICHAEL TORKE, composer

anything from whale and dolphin music to the sounds of waterfalls and waves crashing against the shore.

Try sound therapy to relieve tension and relax your muscles. For a three-minute relaxation, make a long O (as in ocean) or Ah (as in harp) sound. This helps get rid of any thoughts cluttering your mind.

Once you've chosen your sound, lie down quietly, taking even, deep breaths. Try to clear your head. Just let the music wash over you. Your heart rate should lower, your metabolism drop, your eyelids droop…and you're asleep.

42. Say yes to yoga

**Breathing exercises and moves that put
you in the right frame of mind for sleep.**

Once you're regularly practicing yoga, you'll
fall asleep in a shorter time – mainly because your body and mind are
more relaxed. The quality of your sleep will improve and you may
even need less sleep.

By learning how to slow your rate of breathing, you shed yourself of
the day's stresses. Sit or stand where you can see a clock. Put your
hands on your lower ribs and count the number of times you
breathe in and out normally in one minute. Then breathe slightly
faster than usual and count the
breaths that you take in one
minute. Take a break to calm your
breathing, then repeat the exercise,
this time trying to breathe much
more slowly than you normally do.
With practice, you should be able
to slow your rate of breathing to as
few as six breaths a minute – the
usual rate during meditation.

Here's an idea for you

Try 2-1 breathing. Gently slow down
the rate of exhalation until you exhale
for twice as long as you inhale. Don't
try to fill or empty the lungs completely
– you are simply changing the rhythm
of your breath. Your breath should flow
smoothly, evenly and continuously.
When you've mastered it take 8 breaths
lying on your back, 16 breaths on your
right side and 32 on your left side.

103

Defining idea

'Tension is who you think you should
be. Relaxation is who you are'
CHINESE PROVERB

Now try some calming poses. The
child's pose will probably make you
want to drop off immediately.
Kneel down and sit on your feet
with your heels pointing outward
Your knees should be separated,
about the width of your hips. Place your forehead on the floor, then
bring your arms alongside your body, palms turned upward. Stay for
about three minutes. To come up from the child's pose, lengthen the
front of your body then inhale as you lift from your tailbone, pressing
down and into your pelvis

Finally, do the corpse pose. Lie on your back, with your feet spread
about 18 inches apart, your hands about 6 inches from your sides,
palms up. Let your thighs, knees and toes turn outward. Close your
eyes and breathe deeply. Then first tense then relax each part of your
body in turn, working up from your feet to your head.

43. Ommmmm...

**Use meditation to rid yourself of
information overload and clear your head
for bed**

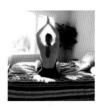

Fans say that meditating helps you to rise above everyday niggles
and sort out what's important to you. Do it regularly, and blood
pressure will fall and levels of your stress hormones will plummet as
will your blood levels of lactic acid, which is associated with anxiety.

Wearing loose clothing sit comfortably with your back straight, either
in a chair or on the floor, with your eyes closed, breathing deeply.
When you breathe bring your
breath right down to your navel
and, as you exhale, let go of any bad
feelings and feel the day's stresses
and worries drift away. Tell yourself
that with each breath you're
becoming more and more relaxed.
The more you practice, the better
you'll get at reaching a state of total
calm. Aim for two 20-minute
sessions a day – ideally once before
breakfast and once in the evening.

Here's an idea for you

Sit comfortably with your spine
reasonably straight. Allow your eyes
to rest downward, not focused on
anything. Without closing your eyes
completely, let your eyelids drop to a
level that feels relaxed and comfortable.
Continue gazing down. You may notice
your breathing gradually becoming more
rhythmic. It's okay to let your attention
drift a bit. If your eyes become very
heavy then let them close.

There are three main different types of meditation:

■ When practising *transcendental meditation*, you repeat a mantra to yourself to prevent distracting thoughts from entering your mind and allow you to gradually relax and release stress. The idea is to reach a passive state where thoughts, images, and feelings pass through your consciousness almost unnoticed.

■ In *mindfulness meditation* all your thoughts and feelings come and go but you don't react to them. Think about each part of your body from head to toe. As you let go of thoughts or images associated with each body part, the body part lets go, too, thus releasing much of its tension. It's also great for cramps, restless legs syndrome and any other pain that could be keeping you awake.

■ *Breath meditation* involves focusing on breathing in and breathing out. Concentrating on something as basic as the breath helps to clear your mind.

44. Herb power

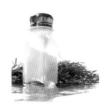

How herbal medicines can help you sleep again.

Certain herbs can help restore proper levels of the sleep-promoting hormone serotonin, while others work by triggering your brain's calming chemicals. Stick to the recommended doses as some herbs can be pretty potent. Alternatively, consult a professional, accredited herbalist.

Chamomile has a sedative effect, and unlike some herbs it's safe for pregnant and breastfeeding women. Put it in your bath in the evening or make a calming tea by adding one teaspoon of the flower to boiling water and steeping for 5–10 minutes.

Hops dried and used to fill a pillow are a traditional remedy for sleeplessness and nervous conditions. You can also buy freeze-dried extract in capsule form.

Here's an idea for you

Buy lavender seeds (lavandula angustifolia) – and plant them indoors on trays until they're ready to be replanted in a pot, windowbox or the garden. As soon as the plants flower, cut the leaves from the stems, tie in loose bunches and leave suspended in a warm dry place until completely dry. Store in an airtight jar. Then prune your lavender plant, ready for next year.

Defining idea

'And still she slept an azure-lidded sleep, In blanched linen, smooth, and lavender'd'
JOHN KEATS

Lavender will help you deal with stress-related insomnia. Make a calming tincture by steeping it in vodka for a month, then straining. Take a teaspoonful three times a day until your tension lifts. Make a sachet of lavender to leave under your pillow at night.

Lemon balm is a sedative. Add 2–3 teaspoons of the dried herb to a cup of freshly boiled water and let it steep for 5–15 minutes for a soothing tea that actually tastes nice too.

Valerian decreases the time it takes to get to sleep and reduces nighttime waking. Put 2–3 droppersful of tincture made from fresh valerian roots (or 1–2 teaspoons of dried valerian root) in hot water for a bedtime drink. Take no more than one cup a day – too much can cause headaches.

St. John's Wort can help relieve chronic insomnia and mild depression when they're due to an imbalance in brain chemistry. It's most commonly taken in capsule form.

45. The sweetest pill

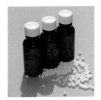

The amazing power of homeopathy.

Ideally you should consult a homeopath to
ensure you take the correct remedy for your symptoms and your
personality type. The remedies are unbelievably specific and can
take into account everything from how tall you are, whether you're
an irritable person or an organiser to whether you've got a good
memory or have a sense of humour. You normally take a remedy an
hour before going to bed for up to 14 days. And if you wake up in
the night and can't get back to sleep, you can repeat the dose. Here
are a few of the more common remedies:

- Nux vomica is for when you wake up around 3 or 4 in the
  morning because you've eaten
  too much the night before or
  had too much alcohol. It suits
  mainly men, competitive types,
  people who are critical but
  can't take criticism from others
  and those who like rich fatty
  food.

Here's an idea for you

If you buy over-the-counter remedies,
log the effects of each remedy you try
in a homeopathy diary. Take only one
remedy at a time and move on to the
next remedy after a few weeks if you're
not happy with the results.

- Pulsatilla is for when you're restless in the early hours of sleep and just can't get comfortable. It suits mainly women, good natured and emotional types, those who prefer sweet food.
- Arnica is for when your bed feels too hard and you are overtired and fidgety. It suits imaginative people and those who put off going to the doctor.
- Lycopodium is for when your mind is active before bed and you're unable to get rid of thoughts about work. You dream a lot and wake up around 4 in the morning. It suits people who are tall and lean, dislike change and are prone to exaggeration.
- Arsenicum is for when you wake up between midnight and 2 in the morning feeling restless and worried. It suits a person who has strong ideas, is attentive to detail and likes everything in its place.
- Rhus tox is for when you can't sleep and feel a need to walk about, or you suffer from restless legs syndrome. It suits those who are lively and anxious at night.

46. It makes scents

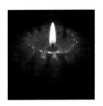

The right aromatherapy oils can relax the mind and body, control stress, relieve pain and beat insomnia.

For a quick and easy way to prepare your body for sleep, you can't beat an aromatherapy bath. Your bath should be warm enough to relax aching muscles and ease tension, but not too hot as this will make the oils evaporate more quickly. A little milk or vodka in the bath will help the oils disperse. Opt for oils that have a relaxing rather than invigorating aroma. For massage always dilute essential oils in a carrier oil such as sweet almond or grapeseed as they'll burn your skin if applied neat. The ideal strength is five to six drops of essential oil to one tablespoon of carrier oil. Always do a patch test before massaging into your skin.

Geranium strengthens the adrenal glands which work overtime when you're stressed. Combine with rosemary for maximum impact. Add a few drops to your bath or listen to some music and put some drops in an oil burner.

Here's an idea for you

Give your partner an aromatherapy massage – then ask for one in return. Get your partner to lie down on his front – either in bed or on the floor with a towel underneath. Add a few drops of chamomile or rose into a light carrier oil, then massage them into his back using circling and kneading movements.

Defining idea

'There must be quite a few things that a hot bath won't cure, but I don't know many of them'
SYLVIA PLATH, *The Bell Jar*

Lavender is the oil most often used for sleep problems as it helps reduce stress, anxiety and depression. Sprinkle a couple of drops on a tissue and inhale or, after a long, hard day put a few drops on your pillow to aid sleep.

Ylang ylang is an aphrodisiac and a sedative too so if the sex doesn't relax you the calming properties of this oil will. Add a couple of drops in a vaporiser for a soothing aroma.

Chamomile calms the central nervous system and induces sleep. It's also a gentle antidepressant and stress reliever. Add a few drops of the oil to your bath.

47. Get to the point

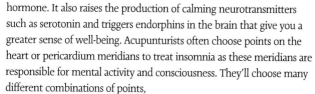

How acupuncture could work for you.

Acupuncture has been shown to lower anxiety and increase levels of melatonin – your key sleep hormone. It also raises the production of calming neurotransmitters such as serotonin and triggers endorphins in the brain that give you a greater sense of well-being. Acupuncturists often choose points on the heart or pericardium meridians to treat insomnia as these meridians are responsible for mental activity and consciousness. They'll choose many different combinations of points, however, depending on the cause of your insomnia – be it restless legs syndrome, headaches or any other pain that's keeping you up at night. Once they've selected your acupuncture points, the needles are quickly inserted. As few as 1 or 2 or as many as 20 or more needles may be used.

Here's an idea for you

Try accupressure on yourself. Press in hard circular motions for up to three minutes. To calm an overactive mind press on the small finger side of the wrist crease in the hollow just below the bone near the outer edge of the wrist. To relax press on the inside of your wrist on the midpoint of the crease. To relieve tension press half a thumb width above your hairline at the front of your head on the centre line.

If done properly you shouldn't feel much when acupuncture needles are inserted – the needles are very fine and pass easily through the skin. You might get a dull or heavy feeling around the needle – this just means the treatment's working. The needles are usually left in for 15–30 minutes. And you'll probably need 6–10 treatments once a week before it works. Regular maintenance sessions can keep your stress levels in check and stop your sleep problems coming back.

Make sure your acupuncturist is qualified and is a member of a recognised professional body. Some medical doctors, nurses and physiotherapists also practice acupuncture. They may have done full acupuncture training or just a weekend course for a specific type of acupuncture such as pain relief, so always check qualifications and don't be afraid to ask about training and experience.

48. Wakey wakey!

Alarm clock or not? The best option for a good night's sleep.

If you wake up naturally, the light of dawn signals your body clock to release your wake-up hormones. An alarm clock obviously interferes with this natural process and allows you to wake up when it's convenient to you. In the moderns world it's not always practical to wake up naturally, so what can you do?

Ideally you should wake up just before your alarm clock goes off – that shows you've had enough sleep. Make sure the alarm clock you choose wakes you up how you want to.

■ Natural alarm clocks simulate sunrise and gradually become lighter and lighter over half an hour, so that you can wake up naturally whenever it suits you. This gradual lightening triggers your body to release all the wake-up hormones. The idea is you'll wake up more refreshed and in a better mood and have more energy all day. There's normally a back-up-beeper for

Here's an idea for you

Train yourself to wake up at a certain time. You've probably done it before when you've had to get up for something important. Tell yourself the night before that you need to wake up at a certain time and after a few nights, it will happen.

heavy sleepers and some even have a sunset go-to-sleep facility where the light slowly fades to darkness – ideal for young children or shift workers.

- Tailor made alarm clocks allow you to record your own wake-up music. Choose your favourite track of the moment or record other sounds.
- Alarm clocks with fade in facility have music which gets gradually louder so you wake up more gently.
- Talking alarm clocks start chatting to you after the alarm goes off. To turn it off you can say 'alarm off' or simply shake it.
- Shaking alarm clocks shake the bed to wake up. If that doesn't work, the flashing lights come on. Sounds like waking up to an erupting volcano to me, but it may work for you.

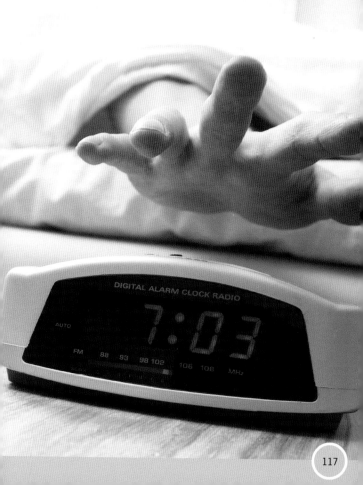

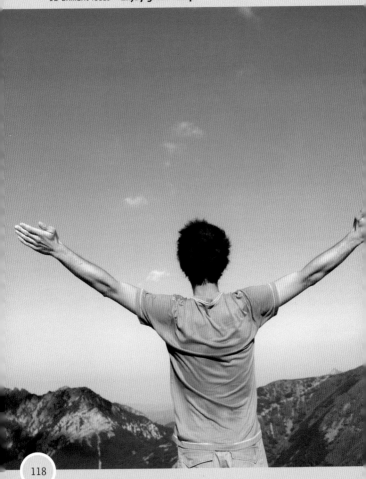

49. Wake-up stretches

This simple stretch routine will get your muscles ready for the day and give you time to wake up properly, clear your head and lift your spirits.

- While lying on your back in bed reach your arms over your head as far as you can, and push your legs as far as they'll go. Hold this stretch for three deep breaths and release, letting your body relax into your bed.
- Sit on the edge of your bed and slump your body over your legs. Starting from your lower back, slowly roll to a sitting position, rolling your shoulders back and looking straight ahead. Slowly roll back down to a slump.
- On all fours on your bedroom floor arch your back as high as possible. Repeat the movement slowly 12–15 times.
- Stand next to a wall, facing sideways, your feet about hip-width apart. Without bending your knees, lean slightly forward as far as you can without tipping or letting your heels come off the floor. Then tilt backward without lifting your toes. Still

Here's an idea for you

Why not brave a cold shower?! Bathing in cold water can boost circulation and increase energy levels – take a three minute hot shower followed by 40–60 seconds of cold water. Repeat three times if you dare.

Defining idea

'I exercise every morning without fail. One eyelid goes up and the other follows.'
PETE POSTLETHWAITE, actor

keeping your feet flat on the floor, sway to the left and then to the right as far as possible.

■ Stand straight, holding a table or chair for balance. Take 3 seconds to bend each knee, trying to get your calf as close to the back of your thigh as possible. Hold, then lower your leg over 3 seconds.

■ Stand next to the wall and face sideways. Slowly raise your right knee over 3 seconds, bringing it as close to your chest as possible. Don't bend at the waist or hips. Hold for a second or two, then lower your leg over 3 seconds. Repeat with your left leg.

■ Stand straight, holding a table or chair for support. Slowly lift your left leg 6 to 12 inches to the side; without bending your knee or upper body. Hold. Slowly lower, and repeat on your right side.

50. Breakfast boosters

Set yourself up for the day with an early morning pick-me-up.

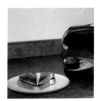

Breakfast can provide up to a quarter of your daily intake of certain vitamins and minerals – including vitamin C, which helps you drop off more easily at night, and the vital B vitamins that make your sleep hormones. Eating a good breakfast means you're less likely to overeat for the rest of the day – particularly important in the evening when a big meal could disrupt your sleep.

When you sleep, your metabolism slows down, but you still need a constant supply of energy in the form of glucose to keep your body and brain ticking over. Glucose is stored in your liver but, because it's not being replaced while you're asleep, your levels are pretty low when you wake up. Your brain needs a new supply to kick-start it into action again.

Here's an idea for you

Make your own muesli. Mix together a handful of oatflakes with your favourite dried fruits, nuts and shaved coconut. Add fruit and yoghurt to plain cereals or mix chopped nuts such as peanuts, hazelnuts or walnuts into porridge.

Defining idea

'All happiness depends on a leisurely breakfast'
JOHN GUNTHER, novelist

By eating breakfast as soon as you can, you rev-up your metabolism and replenish the glucose you lost overnight, providing instant fuel for your brain to function throughout the day. People who eat breakfast perform better mentally and verbally and concentrate better than those who don't. It can boost energy for at least two hours – unlike a big lunch which can lead to an afternoon dip.

Go for a high carbohydrate, low fat meal with plenty of fibre, all washed down with a glass of orange or grapefruit juice or fruit tea. Good ones to try are:

- a bowl of fruit salad, topped with yoghurt and a good sprinkling of muesli;
- a bowl of porridge, topped with chopped banana;
- a bagel with low fat cream cheese and pineapple slices;
- two slices of wholemeal toast with marmite or peanut butter;
- Shredded wheat cereal with skimmed milk and a banana.

51. The joy of Zzzz

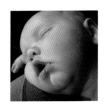

Here are just some of the benefits of getting your full quota of sleep.

Good looks You can spend a fortune on expensive skin creams and watch your diet, but you need your sleep for youthful looking skin. Harmful free radicals – which can lead to premature ageing – are scavenged and cell damage is repaired. And those dark circles around the eyes will be a thing of the past.

Good mood Many of the neurotransmitters in the brain that regulate sleep also regulate mood, which is why sleep deprivation is associated with mood swings. Neurotransmitters, which carry messages to the brain need to be replenished during sleep. When they are, your spirits will be high.

Reduced stress If you get in the habit of writing down your worries – and possible solutions – at least once a week you won't go to bed with a suitcase full of concerns. When you get a good night's sleep you're better able to cope with everyday events so you don't get so affected by stress.

Here's an idea for you

Make a list of everything that improved the quality of your sleep – from lavender essential oil in your bath to visualising a relaxing beach scene. If you start getting sleepless nights again you can refer to your notes.

Defining idea

'Sleep is that golden chain that ties health and our bodies together'
THOMAS DEKKER, playwright

Weight loss Sleep loss interferes with the secretion of cortisol, a hormone that regulates appetite. When your cortisol levels are out of whack, you can feel hungry even if you've had enough to eat. Carbohydrates also metabolise slower when you're sleep-deprived, causing sugars to linger in the blood and jack up insulin production, which increases the storage of body fat.

Less illness Sleep helps your body fight infection because your immune system releases a sleep-inducing chemical while fighting a cold or an infection. Sleep also helps the body conserve energy and other resources that the immune system needs to mount an effective attack.

Mental sharpness When you're sleeping well, you'll be able to concentrate on what people are saying, your memory will return and you'll be able to think more clearly.

52. Quirky questions

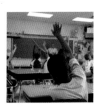

Here are the answers to some of those niggling questions you've always had about sleep but didn't know who to ask.

What's the longest amount of time someone has gone without sleep?
The record is 18 days, 21 hours, 40 minutes after which the record holder reported hallucinations, paranoia, blurred vision, slurred speech and memory and concentration lapses.

How loud is the loudest snore?
One British snoring champion had a 92 decibel snore – louder than a pneumatic drill. Needless to say, his long suffering wife is deaf in one ear.

Can you sleep with your eyes open?
Many parents claim their babies sleep with their eyes open or partially open. Adults can take cat naps with their eyes open without being aware of it and sleepwalkers are technically asleep even though they have their eyes open and appear to be awake.

Do we sleep longer than other animals?
Humans sleep on average around three hours less than other primates such as chimps, rhesus monkeys, squirrel monkeys and

Defining idea

*'If there are no stupid questions, then
what kind of questions do stupid
people ask? Do they get smart just in
time to ask questions?'*
SCOTT ADAMS, US cartoonist

baboons, all of whom sleep for
10 hours.

Can you sleep standing up?
No – you'd fall down as soon as
your muscles relaxed. To stay
standing you have to keep certain
muscles tense, and to control these
muscles you have to be conscious. Horses have a system of tendons
and ligaments that hold them in the standing position while their
muscles relax. So they can lie down or stand up to sleep.

How long do dreams last?
Most dreams last as long as REM sleep – about 20 minutes each. And
they're in real time – that means if you're dreaming about having a
bath it's going to take about the same time as it does in real life.

Is it possible to not dream?
Most people dream, but just don't remember them. Patients treated
for depression have little or no dreaming sleep while they're taking
antidepressants. Their mental health improves and there are no bad
psychological side effects such as loss of memory. This shows that
dream sleep may not be so critical to memory as some people have
previously thought.

This book is published by Infinite Ideas, creators of the acclaimed **52 Brilliant Ideas** series. If you found this book helpful, there are other titles in the **Brilliant Little Ideas** series which you may also find of interest.

brilliant ideas

- **Be incredibly creative**
- **Catwalk looks**
- **Drop a dress size**
- **Enjoy great sleep**
- **Find your dream job**
- **Get fit!**
- **Heal your troubled mind**
- **Healthy children's lunches**
- **Incredible sex**
- **Make your money work**
- **Perfect romance**
- **Raising young children**
- **Relax**
- **Seduce anyone**
- **Shape up your bum**
- **Shape up your life**

For more detailed information on these books and others published by Infinite Ideas please visit www.infideas.com.

See reverse for order form.

Qty	Title	RRP
	Be incredibly creative	£5.99
	Catwalk looks	£5.99
	Drop a dress size	£5.99
	Enjoy great sleep	£5.99
	Find your dream job	£5.99
	Get fit!	£5.99
	Heal your troubled mind	£5.99
	Healthy children's lunches	£5.99
	Incredible sex	£5.99
	Make your money work	£5.99
	Perfect romance	£5.99
	Raising young children	£5.99
	Relax	£5.99
	Seduce anyone	£5.99
	Shape up your bum	£5.99
	Shape up your life	£5.99

Add £2.49 postage per delivery address

Final TOTAL

Name: ....

Delivery address: ....

....

....

E-mail:.............................Tel (in case of problems):

By post Fill in all relevant details, cut out or copy this page and send along with
a cheque made payable to Infinite Ideas. Send to: Brilliant Little Ideas, Infinite
Ideas, 36 St Giles, Oxford OX1 3LD. **Credit card orders over the telephone**
Call +44 (0) 1865 514 888. Lines are open 9am to 5pm Monday to Friday.

Please note that no payment will be processed until your order has been dispatched. Goods are
dispatched through Royal Mail within 14 working days, when in stock. We never forward personal
details on to third parties or bombard you with junk mail. The prices quoted are for UK and RoI
residents only. If you are outside these areas please contact us for postage and packing rates.
Any questions or comments please contact us on 01865 514 888 or email info@infideas.com.